Welcoming an Unwelcome Guest

Marisa Van Staden

Published by Marisa Van Staden, 2024.

WELCOMING AN UNWELCOME GUEST

First edition. March 9, 2024.

ISBN: 979-8224666690

Written by Marisa Van Staden.

Dedication

I dedicate this book to our two daughters, who kept me motivated to keep on fighting the cards that life has played for me, keeping me mentally strong to keep on walking, they both don't know how much they inspired me to keep my willpower and do not give up with life going on all around me, just keep on living.

Gratitude

Of course, there is so many people deserving so much more than a plain "thank you", as that's something you say to someone bringing you coffee. Close family: Parents, expecially my mother and Chat396, who provided me with better wording, spelling and grammer. Our kids, for keeping me motivated through this over the years. Siblling, God mother, Aunts (lots of them). Friends, Pastor, Spouse, for believing in me through it all, no matter how hard the cards are. Draft2Digital for giving possibility to publish my book. So many helped me in their own way, some without even knowing.

CHAPTER 1
MEETING THE UNWELCOMED GUEST

Round and around I go, gliding effortlessly on the ice, revelling in the sweet thrill of being sixteen! It's another one of my pre-exam rituals—something most of my classmates would shy away from, gripped by nerves. But me? I refuse to acknowledge that fear and stress even exist. At sixteen, I possess all the knowledge and wisdom I think I'll ever need. It's hard for me to grasp why anyone would be afraid; to me, the very idea of fear seems absurd! Life's a breeze—why can't they see that? For every problem, there's a solution. So, why focus on the problem when you could be finding the way through it? Chase after your rainbow, and you'll eventually reach it; as for the pot of gold at the end, well, that's up to you to find. With a motto like this, how can anything be impossible to face? Aim for the moon, and even if you miss, you'll still find yourself among the stars.

But now, I know that health and wealth are just as crucial as success. Some things, no matter how much money you have, cannot be bought. My mother's wise words finally make sense. As a teenager, when our family faced financial hardships, I thought I had the answers. I won a printer-scanner in a school competition and swapped it for school fees (yes, I really did that!). I found weekend work washing cars to help with family expenses—every obstacle seemed temporary, and everything had a solution. Even life itself is temporary (there's that teenage wisdom again!).

Moving to my own flat for university in a new town, I thought I had everything figured out. Alone in a big city, with only my mom's close friend nearby and the rest of my family cities away—my parents working abroad in another African country—I was free. Free to do whatever I wanted. So naturally, I started with the essentials: exploring every local club and pub. I even began hypnotherapy sessions, determined to overcome my speech impediment. Though the stuttering eased, it didn't disappear entirely, but I never let it stop me from living life to the fullest.

One night, while visiting my brother in our hometown, I decided to go to a bar with a high school friend. And then it happened: that fateful moment described in movies and whispered in old wives' tales, when "you just know." In an instant, I locked eyes with someone—a gaze that seemed to capture my entire life story: past, present, and future, all at once. I thought, "Oh, come on, not now! I'm busy owning the dance floor!"

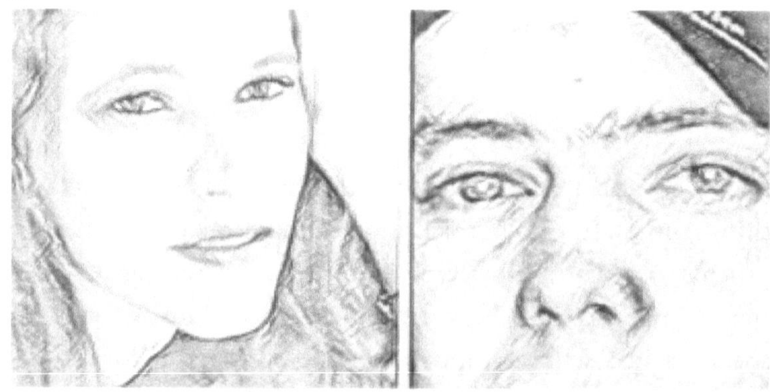

This momentous occasion called for another solution. I decided to move back home, drop out of university, find work, and continue my studies online. This is exactly what I did. Everything was still going well from my perspective, and I believed I could still reach my goals, even as

I fell deeply in love. The next thing that took me by surprise was having two daughters in two years and then getting married. I know it should have been the other way around, but these were the cards life dealt me, so I accepted it and moved forward, adapting as I went.

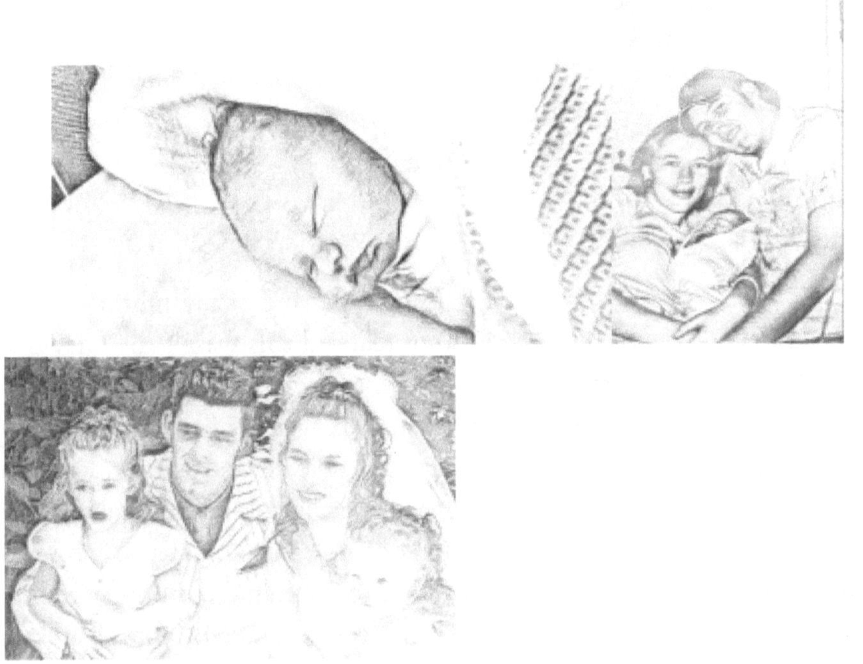

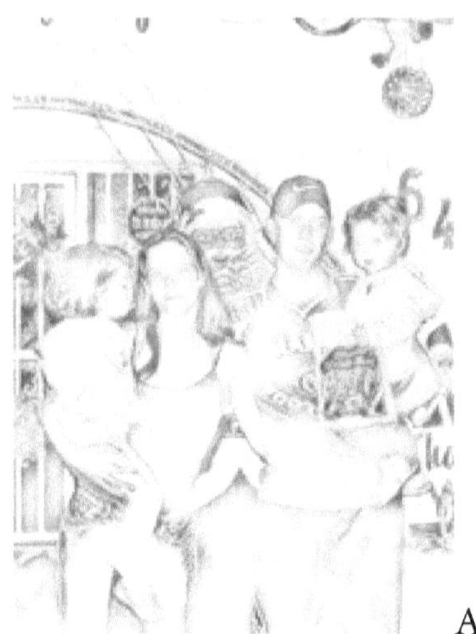

After the sad passing of my mother-in-law and just six weeks of marriage, I soon realized this wasn't the fairy-tale I had foolishly envisioned for myself. Despite being in a good, stable relationship for seven years, it took just six weeks of marriage for me to conclude that I couldn't see it through. Please don't misunderstand me; we both had our faults and made mistakes. But, as usual, I went for the easy solution. Life had always come easily for me, so why not now? I moved out, relocated to another town, found temporary respite with my mother's cousin and his family, then secured a job and a place for myself, my girls, and my dog, Pepper. We settled close to my new job, and I started enjoying a young adult lifestyle. Everything was going smoothly according to my grand plan, to the extent that my ex-husband and I walked out of divorce court joking like old friends, although we still had the occasional telephone fight. Little did I know, I would always love him.

Starting my career in the big city at a resin wholesaler, I loved the city's busy vibe, and even traffic jams didn't faze me. However, after two months, I found the commute to and from work tedious and draining. So, I found a job closer to home, considering it the obvious solution, as it gave me more time for my part-time studies and allowed me to earn extra income through stock market investments. But my mainstay and support were always my parents, who helped me emotionally and financially when my investments didn't yield the expected returns in the anticipated timeframe. Perhaps it was another one of those unrealistic dreams and hopes.

I worked from eight to five, cared for the girls until their bedtime at around 8 or 9 p.m., then worked on my investment portfolio until midnight, only to wake up at around 3 a.m. to keep up with my studies before getting ready for work and taking the girls to daycare. This routine repeated itself for over a year. But I was determined to succeed on my own. With extra vitamins and caffeine boosts, I convinced myself I could make it through another day. Just another two or three years, and I'd be set—almost there!

Determination burned inside me as I focused entirely on where my path was leading. Even though I had gone through rough patches before, I knew I was on my way and strong enough to succeed. Life could throw anything at me, and I had proven that I could fall and still conquer.

I enjoyed a restaurant meal with my parents after the finalization of my divorce. They were home from abroad for two weeks before returning to their jobs. The feeling of being close to completing a puzzle, of finalizing a well-planned path I couldn't stray from, was ever-present. I neglected to consider the reality of what I was doing to others—my daughters only saw their father on occasional set terms, even though, at their young age, they were unlikely to understand any of the proceedings.

All that mattered to me was reaching my goals, being successful, and earning the highest possible salary. Seeing others, especially my ex, struggling and falling by the wayside didn't affect me. In my mind, it was simply a fact of life: if opportunities weren't served to you on a silver platter, you could always pick up the pace and still make your dreams and goals come true.

Returning to my well-ordered life, the company I worked for installed a pepper-gas alarm system as a safety measure during strikes at nearby industries. As I was always the first to arrive at the office in the mornings, it became my responsibility to unlock and deactivate the alarm system. Unfortunately, I punched in the wrong deactivation code and got sprayed with pepper gas in the face. I shook it off after a few minutes and carried on with my day as usual.

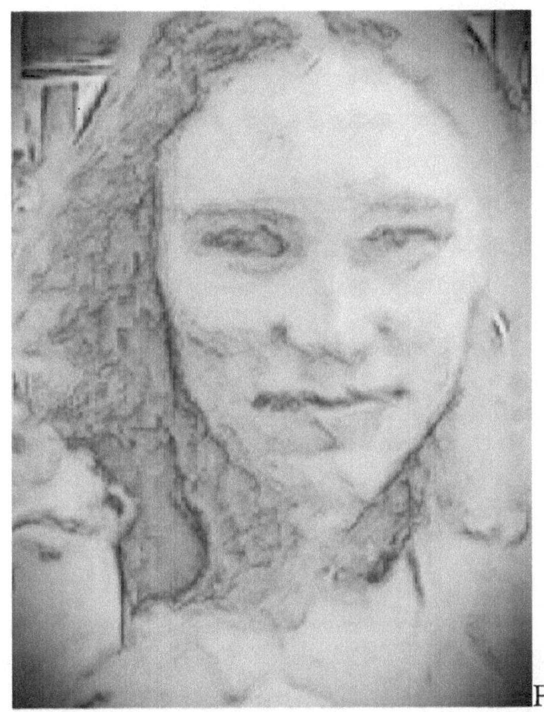

From that day forward, I got sprayed in the face with pepper gas on average twice a week because my right hand would shake, causing me to enter the wrong code by accident. This was surprising, coming from a woman who thrived on solving mathematical problems and had an excellent memory, especially when it came to recalling complex sequences of numbers. For crying out loud, I could remember the registration numbers of vehicles we drove ten years ago; I could recite from memory not only my own but also my daughters', my ex's, and my parents' identity numbers, as well as their telephone numbers! But I didn't feel any concern about forgetting one measly code or spilling coffee every morning as I carried the cup up the stairs to my office—I'd just start the day with half a cup!

Symptoms gradually worsened to the point where I became extremely confused with numbers, names, codes, and dates. For a woman who used to type at over 80 words per minute with 100% accuracy, declining to only 19 words per minute with 30% accuracy was a glaring red flag. My first step was, of course, to visit my local GP. I was convinced it was a minor issue, and even if it wasn't, I assumed I would be sent for tests to determine the cause of this strange phenomenon. When I was diagnosed with a simple middle-ear infection, the solution seemed straightforward—a course of antibiotics, and everything would be back to normal.

However, the most alarming incident had yet to emerge. I called my father, whose birthday is in May, on the twelfth of September and sang him "Happy Birthday." Although the date was correct, I was way off on the month. This incident raised concerns among my family and friends, spreading like wildfire. My parents booked the first available flight home, my new GP asked what substances I was using that could influence me, and my employer discreetly inquired about the supplements I was taking. My answer was always the same: I only took B vitamins, Omega oil capsules, Bioplus boost, and plenty of coffee.

Still holding onto a strong, positive belief that everything would be fine soon, I went ahead and resigned from my job to have more time to focus on my studies and complete my degree while continuing with my investment venture. I even cancelled my medical aid and life insurance policies, including disability cover, as I was convinced, I would be able to resume my career after 18 months—this time with a degree to my name. How great would that be! Part of my dream was to bring my parents back home permanently and to spend more time with my kids in the meantime. In hindsight, it seems like an illogical decision, but at the time, it felt like a solid plan to fulfil my goals and dreams, creating a perfect life for my daughters and myself. It was just 18 months—I was sure I could manage it, no fear.

But looking back, I realize that when you have a "no-fear" attitude, the "fear" part becomes amplified, and the "no" falls away, becoming merely a descriptive adjective. Without realizing it, I was left with only the fear. During my notice period, a nationwide strike occurred, impacting the industry but not directly affecting the company I worked for. However, it influenced the surrounding areas, starting from the city centre and moving closer to us. All our employees still showed up for work, and we continued our duties as usual. One day, as the strikes drew closer, our MD called on a security company to protect the workforce. Armed guards were placed at all the entrances along our street, and the employees were instructed to leave and get home safely.

My first thoughts were of my children. Driving through the streets out of the industrial area felt safe with the guards present. Armed guards didn't scare me—my father was an ex-army major, and I grew up around armed people. When I arrived at the kids' school, I wanted to calm my nerves, so I sat down in the middle of the sandpit, not thinking about numbers, graphs, or responsibilities—just spending time with my

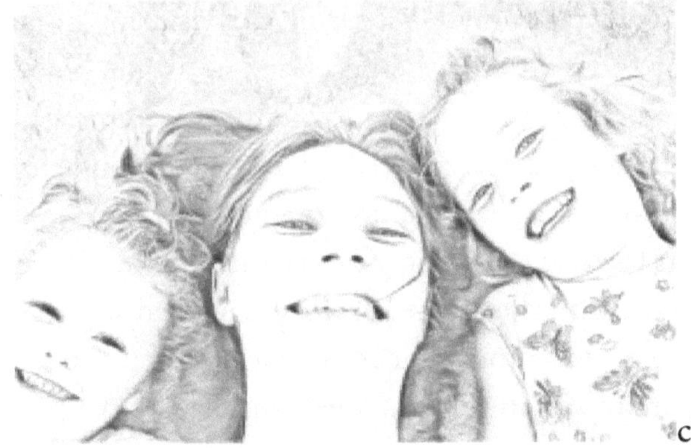

children in my formal

business suit. I noticed a familiar woman walking through the school gate; it was the same lady from that morning who had remarked, "It's a shame to be drunk this early in the morning." I knew she was referring to me, but I couldn't judge her, as I didn't know what was wrong with me either. I probably would have reacted the same way if I had seen a mother dropping off her kids at school and struggling to navigate the stairs or walk in a straight line.

Even though I had no idea what was happening to me, I remember hoping that she would never have to go through the same thing. But what other people thought of me wasn't my concern, not even if I went to the mall with my slippers still on. Strangely, I could still drive, but I couldn't walk a straight line or climb stairs (though, of course, how well I could still drive was questionable, as I had recently scratched my car for the first time). While sitting in the sandpit, I felt a concerned gaze on my back. Turning around, I saw my friend Landi, a teacher at the daycare. She expressed her concern for my health and offered her support if I ever needed it. At this stage, no one believed it was just a middle-ear infection anymore—not me, my parents, my family, friends, or colleagues.

A few days after my parents returned to the country, my mother and I went to another appointment with my GP. During the visit, my mom suggested to the GP that further tests were necessary, as all my blood and urine tests had come back normal, but my symptoms were now at a concerning level. The GP agreed and referred me to a neurologist for further testing, with the earliest available appointment a week away. In the meantime, my parents focused on taking me to calming places. It was during a visit to a restaurant with them that I realized I needed support, not only on stairs but also on escalators. Our conversations often circled back to my health and, more specifically, the question of why the first specialist my GP referred me to a neurologist. My initial thought was that it must be a brain tumour. Perhaps it was fear talking, or maybe I was preparing myself for the worst so that if the news was even slightly better—though still bad—I wouldn't feel as devastated. This way, I could maintain the determination to stand up and fight.

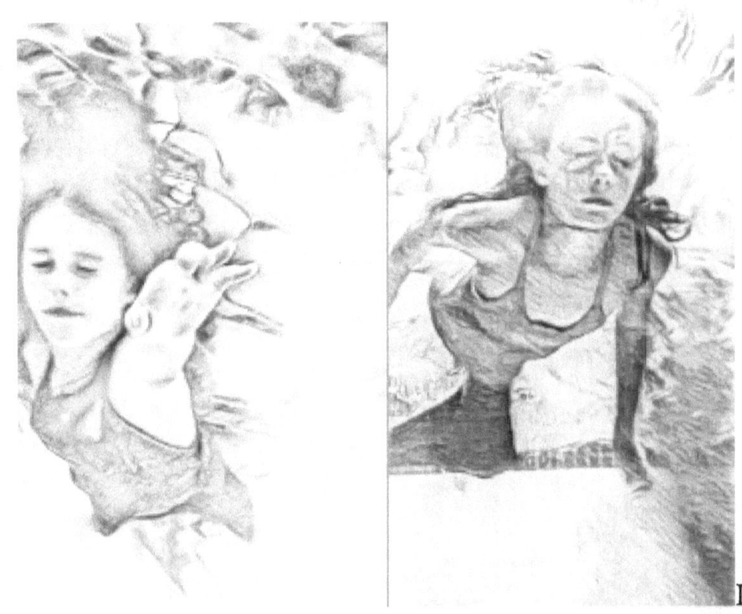

I also continued taking the children to the public swimming pool, as we all loved water-based activities, especially swimming.

While watching the kids enjoy themselves in the pool, I felt a strong urge to experience the calming sensation of water surrounding me. However, I was sure there was no way I could execute a perfect dive into the water; I wasn't even confident about climbing into the pool using the steps. So, for now, I decided to head to the tuck-shop for some coffee instead. As I sat down, I noticed the two tuck-shop attendants observing me. My parents wanted me to sit and relax, but I was determined to make it to the tuck-shop and back. Karin, the older attendant, responded to my order with, "We don't actually sell coffee, but I'll make you some, and my daughter will bring it over." What the heck? I felt my temper rising, but I got up and returned to my parents, where my mom calmed me down.

I realized that my temper was really deteriorating, and I was losing my cool over every little, unnecessary issue. I started to dislike the person I was becoming, unable to control these outbursts. I vividly remember one morning when I went to my upstairs neighbour's apartment at 3:00 a.m. to tell her off for walking around in high heels, which was keeping me from sleeping. This had never bothered me before, but it was an indication of the sleeping disorder that was creeping up on me, and it was the least acceptable symptom of all.

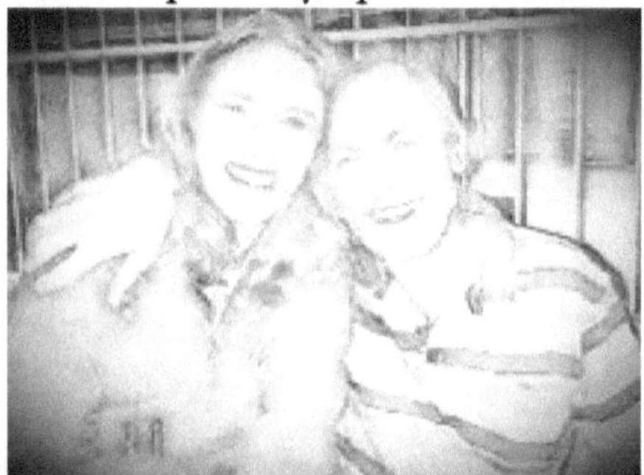

My father accompanied me to the neurologist appointment, where the doctor conducted some simple balancing and reflex tests. For example, I had to walk in a straight line, stand on one leg for a few seconds, and lift both my arms while trying to maintain my balance. Of course, the classic "knee-jerk" test, where a soft hammer is used to hit my bent knee, was part of these assessments. His conclusion: I needed to get an MRI scan. When we asked about what could possibly warrant such a step, the only part of his answer I clearly recall is that he really hopes it's not what he thinks it is but can only give me a definitive answer once the scan results are in. Another week to wait for the scary scan!

During that week, my symptoms continued to manifest as stress, depression, and uncertainty wreaked havoc on my mind. At this point, I couldn't visit the toilet alone or get in and out of the bath without assistance. The question hammering in my brain was: How am I supposed to raise our two girls alone?

I remembered a few weeks earlier, before my parents arrived to support me, when a friend took the girls and me to the seaside for a short vacation. I couldn't walk fast, let alone run, and I was heartbroken when our eldest daughter, only six years old, struggled with the waves breaking on the beach. I couldn't get to her quickly enough to prevent her from going under. Thankfully, a lady nearby rushed in and pulled her to safety. This further undermined my belief that I could take care of our girls.

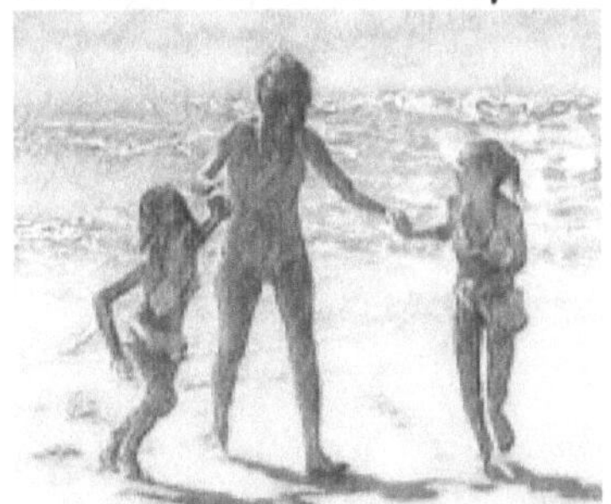

But all my worries, fears, and uncertainties, I kept to myself—no lamenting on social media about lost abilities or confusing, scary symptoms. In fact, I didn't even inform the girls' father, preferring to wait until we had a firm diagnosis and a solution (a timeframe for complete recovery) for the future. My father had to return to work abroad, and he first needed to make time to help me remove the clamps from my hair extensions. My mom managed to get some additional time off so she could stay with me when I needed her most.

The scan date finally arrived, and my mom and I were taken to the hospital by a friend familiar with the area and roads in that city. I tried to prepare myself for the worst-case scenario—that I had a tumour and only weeks to live! —but reasoned that anything better than that would feel far less traumatic.

While changing into a hospital gown and getting ready for the scan, my mind was a whirlwind of what-ifs, and I felt quite sick with anxiety. Fortunately, the nurse taking me to the half-tunnel scanner was a caring and compassionate woman who did her best to calm my fears. She had me lie down on the machine, arranging pillows beneath my knees and against my ears. As she went into a small adjoining room, I could see her observing me through the darkened window. Each calm cycle of the machine took me back to a tranquil moment in my life, the most recent being when my father had removed my hair extensions with pliers before, he went back abroad. Just before I nodded off, the machine would start scanning again, creating a loud noise.

I noticed the nurse's concerned expression as she looked at me, then back at her computer. When she returned to the room, she wouldn't even let me walk back to the dressing room on my own. At that moment, I realized that whatever this was, it was very serious. We spent an hour cooling our heels in the hospital cafeteria while waiting for the scans to be ready. Strangely, I now felt calm, probably because I knew I would have an answer within the next hour or two. With the nurse's solemn look etched in my mind, I prepared myself for the worst-case scenario.

My mother went into the neurologist's office with me. As he placed one of my scans on the lighted whiteboard and began explaining the technical image before us, I got lost in the Milky Way picture of my brain. I glanced at my mother next to me; she was clasping her hands together but couldn't hide their shaking. She was staring straight at the doctor, swallowing tears. I immediately concluded: Okay, this is it; I have a few weeks left. But I couldn't comprehend what the problem was. The neurologist suggested we go into the garden to assimilate the news and to come back to his office when we felt ready to discuss it further.

Outside on the sidewalk, my mother and her friend were crying, and my mom hugged me tightly. I didn't fully understand what we were crying about, but since it must be really bad, I joined in regardless. They then explained to me that I had been diagnosed with multiple sclerosis—something treatable but not curable. I would need to learn to continue life as normally as possible while adjusting to this new reality of limitations and lost abilities. But the greatest news was that I WAS NOT DYING; THERE WAS NO TUMOR! After a quick prayer of thanks and gratitude that it was ONLY multiple sclerosis and not the expected worst-case scenario, I felt a sense of relief. The bottom line was that I could still go on and live with this! To me, this situation was comparable to completing a stage in a digital game, where you receive instructions before entering the next level.

We returned to the neurologist's office, where we received more specific information regarding medication and steps to improve my cognitive abilities, balance, and state of mind through exercise, relaxation, and nutrition. Optimal health in mind and body would allow me to lead a fairly normal life. However, my mind was interpreting all this information to suggest that I was now a vegetable. Then again, being a vegetable must have some advantages, right? Nothing is one hundred percent negative, and somewhere, there's always a sliver of positivity hiding—even if it's small. It's a starting point from which growth can occur if nurtured and treated right. The most burning question at this point was: What was the root cause of this disease in my body? When you can trace something back to its origin, surely, you'll have more weapons and understanding to fight against it. Shockingly, I received an answer that completely baffled me: "Some of us were just designed to self-deconstruct."

Really??!! How on earth could I agree with this statement when it was clear that the good doctor did not know who "constructed" or created us? Needless to say, I never went back to this neurologist. I was admitted to the hospital, where I was put on a cortisone drip and had to endure a lumbar puncture to determine the severity of this disease. Since I had cancelled my medical aid a few weeks before this diagnosis, the financial implications were a significant concern. For the first time in my life—after 26 years of stubborn independence and sole decision-making—I was forced to accept life for what it is and trust that the answers would be provided without my needing to analyze risks, calculate possible outcomes, and compare different scenarios on my own.

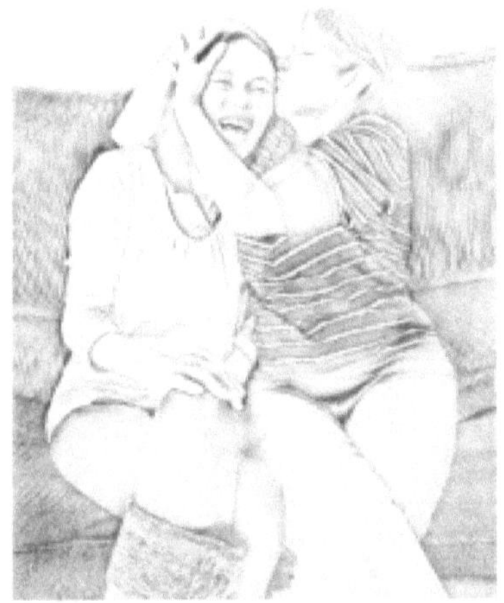

My mother stayed with me during this time, helping me until the sky slowly regained some of its brightness. Transportation for our girls to and from school was arranged, utilizing the support of a teacher and a close friend. Neighbours, family, and friends jumped in to offer assistance wherever and however they could. Thanks to a work loan arranged through my mother's employer, the hospital expenses were fully covered. Without me lifting a finger, everything was being sorted and put in place.

During those first crucial weeks, when preparing meals was difficult due to the extreme heat of pots and stoves and the risk of burning food if I wasn't quick enough, my mother was there. She took over the motherly duties, caring for the girls, cooking meals, and also assisting me with bathing (helping me in and out of the tub and checking the water temperature, just to be on the safe side). I was blessed with a live-in nurse and received an abundance of tender loving care. Looking back after seven years, I'm not sure how I would have coped without that support. Even without being overwhelmed by cash flow problems, I managed to live not "the perfect life," but "my perfect life." Anyone going through that first crucial time of adjusting, adapting, and coming to terms with their new reality needs a lot of understanding, care, and, mostly, unconditional love from those around them. Combining every little act of caring, support, and assistance quickly adds up to a great deal of positivity in a life gone haywire.

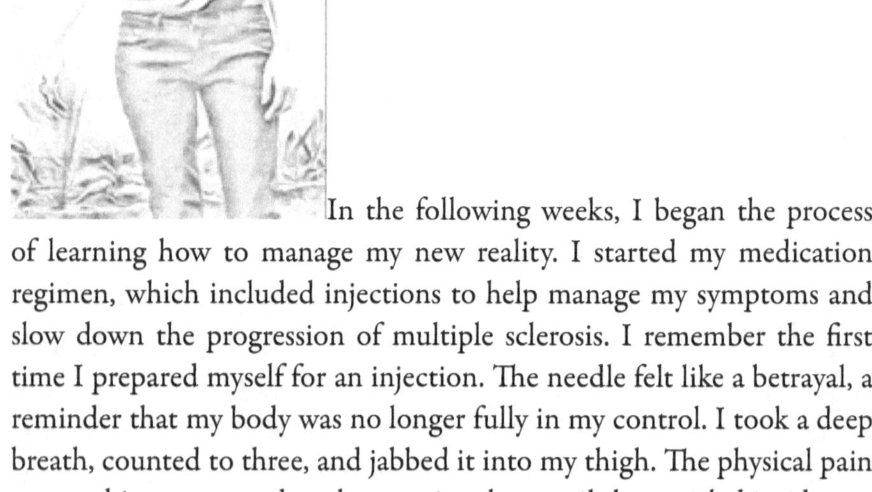

In the following weeks, I began the process of learning how to manage my new reality. I started my medication regimen, which included injections to help manage my symptoms and slow down the progression of multiple sclerosis. I remember the first time I prepared myself for an injection. The needle felt like a betrayal, a reminder that my body was no longer fully in my control. I took a deep breath, counted to three, and jabbed it into my thigh. The physical pain was nothing compared to the emotional turmoil that swirled inside me. I was angry and scared, grappling with the sudden changes in my life.

Support from my family and friends became my lifeline. My mother continued to stay with me, providing both physical help and emotional support. She cooked, cleaned, and took care of the girls while I tried to adjust. My father, though far away, called regularly, offering words of encouragement and love. Friends reached out, inviting me for coffee, sending messages, and checking in to see how I was coping. I had always prided myself on being independent, but now I had to lean on others, and it felt both foreign and freeing.

Therapy sessions became part of my routine as well. I met with a psychologist who helped me navigate the storm of emotions that came with my diagnosis. We discussed my fears, frustrations, and the grief I felt for the life I thought I would have. Each session felt like a step toward reclaiming some of my power. Slowly, I learned to express my emotions rather than bottle them up. It was a relief to share my burdens with someone who understood the weight I was carrying.

I also began to explore physical therapy, which aimed to improve my strength and balance. At first, the exercises were incredibly challenging. Simple tasks that I once took for granted—like standing on one leg or climbing stairs—now felt like monumental feats. I often left sessions feeling exhausted, both physically and mentally. But I also felt a glimmer of hope; each small victory was a reminder that I could adapt and overcome.

One sunny afternoon, I decided to take the girls to the park. I was nervous about how I would manage, but I knew they needed the outing. With my mother by my side for support, we headed to the local playground. I watched the girls laugh and play, their joy infectious. I took a deep breath and decided to join them on the swings. As I sat down, I felt the cool breeze on my face and the weight of my worries lifted, even if just for a moment.

That day was a turning point for me. I realized that while my life had changed drastically, it didn't mean I had to give up on the things I loved. I began to embrace the idea of redefining my life rather than mourning what was lost. I could still create beautiful moments with my girls, even if they looked different than before.

With the support of my family, therapy, and a growing determination, I set small goals for myself. I wanted to be more active, improve my mobility, and create a new routine that included the things that brought me joy. As I adapted to my new normal, I discovered a resilience within me that I never knew existed. Each day was a new opportunity to learn, grow, and find ways to thrive in this uncharted territory.

As weeks progressed, I slowly started to regain some independence. I was enrolled in a rehabilitation program that focused on balance, coordination, and cognitive exercises. Each session was both a challenge and a triumph. I often found myself frustrated with my body, which felt foreign and uncooperative. Yet, amidst the struggle, there were glimmers of hope. I was learning to celebrate small victories: managing to walk a few extra steps without support or recalling a name that had eluded me for days.

The support from family and friends was invaluable. My mother continued to be my rock, helping me navigate through each day. She encouraged me to embrace my new reality, reminding me that it was okay to ask for help. Her presence was a source of comfort, and I found solace in our shared moments, whether it was enjoying a cup of tea or simply sitting together in silence.

As I gradually adjusted to my new routine, I realized how important it was to prioritize self-care. I began to explore mindfulness practices like meditation and gentle yoga. These moments of stillness provided me with clarity, allowing me to connect with my body and mind on a deeper level. I learned to appreciate the present, cherishing the beauty in small things—a blooming flower, a child's laughter, or a warm hug.

Yet, there were still days filled with uncertainty and fear. The questions about my future loomed large, but I found strength in acknowledging them. I was determined to continue my journey, not just for myself but for my daughters. I wanted to show them that resilience is born from adversity and that it's okay to embrace vulnerability.

In the midst of all these changes, I also discovered a newfound passion for writing. Putting my thoughts on paper became a form of therapy. I began journaling my experiences, capturing the highs and lows, the struggles and triumphs. It was liberating to express myself freely, and I hoped that one day, my words could inspire others facing similar challenges.

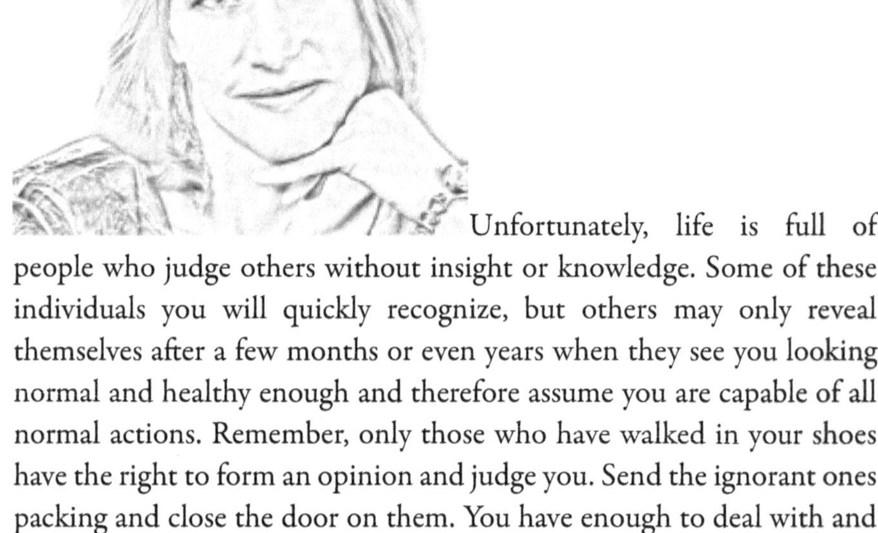

Unfortunately, life is full of people who judge others without insight or knowledge. Some of these individuals you will quickly recognize, but others may only reveal themselves after a few months or even years when they see you looking normal and healthy enough and therefore assume you are capable of all normal actions. Remember, only those who have walked in your shoes have the right to form an opinion and judge you. Send the ignorant ones packing and close the door on them. You have enough to deal with and shouldn't feel obliged to educate those who are judgmental. However, be careful not to become the one acting on assumptions, as this can lead to severe loss without even realizing it at the moment. Logic is not what it used to be!

My first tentative steps into this new reality began with research and gaining perspective. The easiest and most convenient method was to simply talk about it! I made up my mind to be open and forthcoming about my condition, even telling my ex (Jaco) about it. My mom welcomed family, friends, and neighbours, explaining multiple sclerosis to them when they dropped in to offer support. This led to people recalling others with the same condition, and I took contact details whenever possible. Soon, I started connecting with people living with MS in my area, some having been diagnosed many years ago. It quickly became clear to me that every person diagnosed with MS had different symptoms—no similarities or probable causes were found. But I wanted to know what caused this; I wanted to understand the core of what I was up against.

Could it be overwork? The metal used for my hair extension clips? The pepper gas? Genetics? Or does it even exist? I initially thought it might just be physiological, but I wasn't ignoring it, as the proof from the Milky Way image indicated it was real. That's why, if anyone said the words, "It's only in your head!" I could readily agree because, in reality, it is in my head. Most times, they understood the reason for my agreeing differently! But I understood, and that is all that matters in the end.

I started ruling out the probable causes one by one. It couldn't be overwork, as there were people who had also been diagnosed who never worked at a career or had less stressful days with a stable family life. It couldn't be due to caffeine, as I was the only coffee addict. It couldn't be the pepper gas since no one else I spoke to had been sprayed with the same gas (or any gas, for that matter). It couldn't be genetic, as I am the only one in my family ever diagnosed with MS. Therefore, it must be psychological. My theory at this stage was something like a "silent stroke" (if such a thing even existed) or even a severe panic attack, which could explain the Milky Way image. Since the doctors recognized it as multiple sclerosis, I decided to believe it too.

The unwelcome guest took over my brain as its living space, like making up the sleeper couch for unexpected visitors. So, okay, live there, make yourself at home, and let's get to know each other at least.

I came across many possible reasons and unhealthy foods for this condition on Google. Cigarette smoking was obviously the main culprit and was mentioned as detrimental to MS on almost every page I read. I agree it's not a cause, but it definitely worsens the symptoms. Smoking has already been the last thing on my mind since I looked into that "milky way" picture; lighting up another cigarette was no longer an option. Other "symptom intensifiers" I came across online were dairy, sugar, fatty foods, red meat, wheat, etc. I was stumped as to which ones were the most harmful, so I cut all of them from my diet! I replaced them with healthier substitutes as far as possible, but eventually, after about three months, I became really weak and lost a lot of weight. At this stage, my parents took the girls and me on a family vacation, but due to my "healthy diet," I was so weak that I couldn't enjoy it. I was also unable to write my final second-year exams for my B. Com degree. This was heartbreaking because my studies were extremely important to me, and even though I tried extremely hard to be ready in time for those finals, I had to concede defeat. The day before my favourite subject (Maths), I wrote a sentence on a blank piece of paper for my father, asking, "Ag, please Daddy, can I?" He looked at me with a world of sympathy and empathy, knowing how badly I wanted to prove that I still had the ability. He simply replied, "Sorry, not yet," while suppressing his tears. Eventually, I bounced back and promised myself that one day I would get there—I would obtain my degree and put in the hard work necessary to achieve it.

My father prepared a meal, starting with my favourite foods: chicken livers, cauliflower in a white sauce, and maize meal. Slowly, I began incorporating all the forbidden, but delicious, foods back into my diet. My physical strength improved dramatically to the point where I could even do cartwheels with the girls again. Nothing fancy and not a perfect cartwheel, but I did it nonetheless. My mother came home with a tin of decaf coffee and wisely told me to take it on a trial-and-error basis. Eventually, I got all the disallowed foods back into my diet, except for sugar in my coffee, as I found that it now spoiled the taste. But anything else with sugar was gladly accepted!

I remember one day when my mother and I sat on the porch, talking about what we had learned so far regarding this condition. She then made a startling but accurate observation: I hadn't stuttered even once since this whole ordeal. It begs the question: Could my stuttering from a young age have been related to Multiple Sclerosis, as speech is one of its known symptoms? Or is it simply that I am now more aware and cautious in my speech because I know it is a symptom? But I didn't really care about the reason for my smooth speech, as long as it worked, and therefore, I am sticking to it!

Driving became the next challenge—an ability I had to work hard to regain. The same applied to typing and writing. I practiced at least one of the three every single day, even if some days it was only for thirty minutes or an hour. What I still cannot understand, to this day, is why I can drive a car, but climbing stairs on my own is beyond me! Although, truthfully, I was only confident driving short distances within the same, familiar neighbourhood—no long distances yet. But that's okay; I'll get there. For now, I am concentrating on baby steps.

Exercising became a regular routine, and by focusing on my legs and core area, I was optimistic that I would get my balance back soon. It actually improved quite a lot! I joined a nearby gym but had difficulty climbing the stairs to the entrance. However, I never missed a session and kept at it until I reached my goals. I could now climb stairs up and down with only the occasional balancing touch on the rails. I realized this is why driving was easier—I was holding onto a steering wheel! With stairs, I only needed to touch the rails. In the absence of rails, our girls would support me and hold my hand. I liked to imagine that we looked like a picture of a caring mom leading her children by the hand, when, in fact, it was the caring kids leading their mom by the hand! But I didn't mind if I looked like an overprotective mom; I was thankful and proud of the girls for their understanding and assistance, making the road to health easier and even fun.

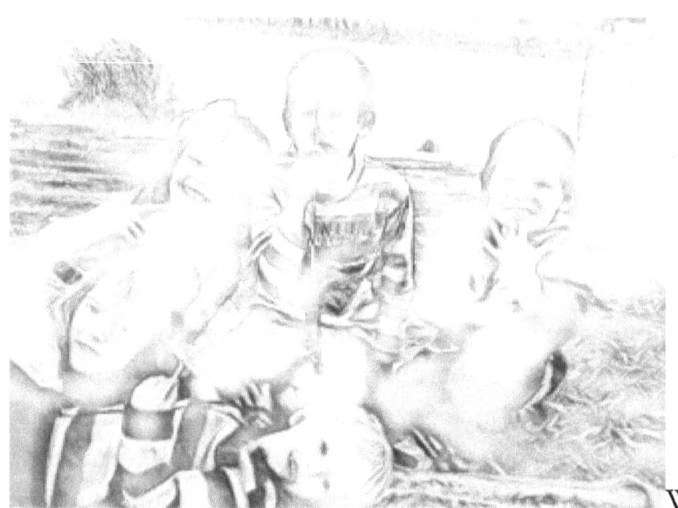

We spent a lot of quality family time together. One of the days I treasure most is when we had a picnic at a lake close to our house, accompanied by my brother, Hekkie, and his family, who came to visit. He is the person always in another town (mostly relatively close to ours), but the first to arrive if I need help. I decided there and then that the lake was the perfect place to come in the mornings after dropping the girls off at school, to jog and meditate. I would then return home, take a quick shower, and pick the girls up from school. I started getting familiar with this guest of mine and liked the new values of life I seemed to have found. Before, they were just normal facts of life. The things I treasured the most before were exam results and studying. During the meditation sessions facing the lake, with my back turned toward the busy morning traffic and sitting at the end of a playground slide, I would conjure up a comic scene in my mind: I pictured my white and red blood cells skating together through my veins, laughing and joking, just having fun together. This meditation naturally ended in prayer. This was when I practiced my ability to use two simple words: "Thank you." These are now the most used words in my vocabulary.

And then the day arrived: I woke up that morning and overheard my mother talking to my dad on the phone. She was telling him to book her a flight back to work. Her exact words were, "She can reason and argue like she used to—she is ready to face circumstances on her own again!"

CHAPTER 2
CALM WATERS

Through my research—talking to people in similar situations, engaging on social media, and exploring health sites online—I quickly understood that Multiple Sclerosis isn't the same for every person. The symptoms vary, as the condition manifests differently in each individual. Another crucial aspect to understand is the various triggers that can lead to a relapse. Time and again, I found that stress and depression play a significant role—just as they do in general life, even for those without medical conditions. Therefore, avoiding these two elements is essential, though it's often easier said than done! Almost everything in life involves some level of stress, even when engaged in a supposedly relaxing hobby. Some hobbies, like gambling, not only increase stress tremendously but can also lead to depression, especially if you encounter financial difficulties. And depression has an even more severe impact on those with Multiple Sclerosis compared to mere stress.

First, pinpoint the elements that cause stress in your life, even if it requires a trial-and-error approach. Create scenarios to anticipate when something might turn into a disaster, and develop the wisdom to abandon unrealistic goals, whether they be financial or emotional. Assess the importance of each goal first—is it something you can live without if it doesn't materialize? Is there an alternative if the goal doesn't come to fruition? Develop a Plan B, C, D... for different possible outcomes before you engage in any challenge, even in relationships. I know it's instinctual to pursue relationships, but for someone with a medical condition, they have the potential to cause stress. If you fail to manage stress, it can eventually lead to depression and trigger a relapse. Keep all possible stress and depression factors out of your life. There's no alternative; you must learn to manage it. Treat each situation as just another speed bump—take it slowly. Too much change too quickly can be detrimental, even if it feels right and good at the time.

With my parents abroad, I had no choice but to manage my life as best as I could, with Pearl, my domestic worker and valued friend, helping to keep the household tasks from overwhelming me. She always ensured I remained as calm as possible. For a few weeks, I drove the children to school in the mornings while still in my pyjamas, as the electronic gates of our complex meant I didn't have to get out of the car. So, it didn't matter that I wasn't dressed in casual clothes—no one could see me!

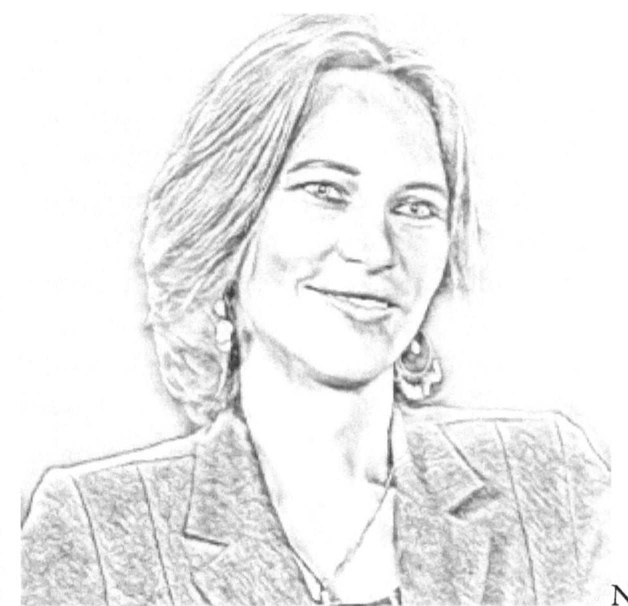

Not even two months after my mother left, I suffered my first relapse. The symptoms included short-term memory loss, slurred speech, and impaired coordination. One peculiar phenomenon was that the stuttering, which I had struggled with all my life, suddenly disappeared after I was diagnosed and began treatment for Multiple Sclerosis! People close to me were used to my speech impediment, so it didn't affect our conversations. However, it was impossible for me to read aloud in class at school, and meeting new people was a stressful experience, impacting my social life. I underwent speech therapy and psychological treatment, which helped to some extent but didn't perfect my speech. Hypnotherapy had a better outcome, but I still couldn't speak as fluently as most people. Speech difficulties are a known symptom of Multiple Sclerosis, and given that I'd stuttered since childhood, it amazed me that none of the professionals addressing my speech problem had ever considered that it might be a neurological issue rather than a psychological one or a bad habit. Since my diagnosis, I can't stutter, even if I try!

I started to explore all the possible causes: Was I simply overworked? Was it the high doses of caffeine? Was it genetic? Could it be the pepper gas? These questions whirled in my mind constantly. Eventually, before they drove me mad, I decided to accept the hand I was dealt. Most days, I live in calm acceptance of the facts, but sometimes I still wonder... One day, I decided to get in my car and search for some peace regarding this whole concept. Shivering—not from the cold, but from the turmoil inside—I set out without knowing my destination. It felt like I wasn't in control of the steering wheel. I saw a billboard advertising a church and found myself stopping in front of its gate. To this day, I don't know why, but I'm grateful I got out of the car. Shaking, shivering, and crying, I made my way to the door. Just as I was about to enter, the pastor came out, on his way to a funeral. He saw me collapsing against the wall and, with concern, took me to his office, where I cried like a baby. He calmed me down by sharing Bible verses, reassuring me that I wasn't being punished, that my Saviour loves me and will be with me every step of the way. He told me to stay close to Him and allow Him to work His miracle.

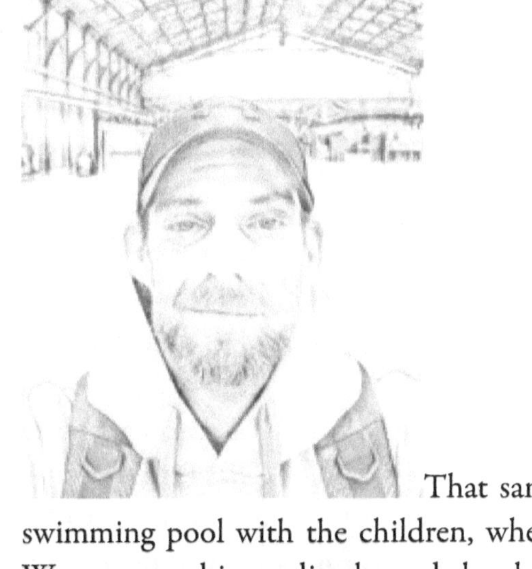

That same afternoon, I returned to the swimming pool with the children, where I got to know Karin better. We connected immediately, and she shared her first impression of me. At first, she thought I must be drunk, but when I approached to order coffee, she realized there was something medically wrong. After that, I visited the pool frequently and began going to church regularly. I also continued my exercise routine and meditation. The thought of my body attacking itself started to fade, and I began seeing myself as normal. I decided to keep this unwelcome guest locked away in a corner; it wouldn't influence me any longer.

A few days later, I had a dream where I ran out of my front door and lost my balance. As I stumbled, a man caught me and pulled me up. I recognized his face, though I couldn't see it clearly. I felt his touch and believed for years that I would recognize my perfect life partner by this touch. I started meeting new people and going on dates, searching for a partner who could walk this path with me. After numerous disappointments, I put the idea to rest, deciding that I would recognize him when he literally caught me as I fell. Only later did I realize that the dream might have symbolized God's presence, guiding me through this journey. The perfect partner indeed! I finally understood the meaning of having Him in our midst as the proactive Saviour we all need—whether we realize it or not, everyone needs Him.

For the following weeks, I focused on finding calm surroundings. I would go jogging next to a lake, even though my steps were like those of a one-year-old learning to run. Afterward, I would go to my favourite spot at the end of the playground slide, where I would sit and meditate, imagining my body cells playing joyfully in my veins. I faced the peaceful ducks on the lake, with my back to the busy road where people hurried for their next pay check. This picture was symbolic: I was forced to turn my back on the rat race and focus on the finer, more important aspects of life that we often take for granted. The most important of these is our health and acknowledging the assistance we need from our Creator.

I concluded that I would need a few months' salary to create a sustainable home business that would allow me to live the calmer lifestyle I envisioned with my daughters and parents once they returned permanently. Making this lifestyle possibly became my goal. I enrolled in an online university and completed my financial degree while searching for employment. However, my job search mainly led to freelance work, helping clients with year-end financials, debtors, creditors, and payroll administration. This flexible work allowed me to spend time with my daughters at the pool or practice piano at the church whenever I needed some calm. I now had the time to prioritize my health, although I still couldn't bring my parents back permanently from abroad. This bothered me, as I believed they were only working overseas to support me financially since I couldn't fully provide for my daughters on my own. They always argued against my opinion, saying they started working abroad long before I needed their help and that I was managing the household in their absence, including handling their salaries and depositing them into various accounts. Imagine—me, who couldn't even walk straight, carrying all that cash in my handbag!

I thought it wise to begin a stress-relief or anti-depressant regimen before returning to the office and corporate environment. I spoke to my GP about it, and he agreed, starting me on the smallest dose of an anti-depressant. Chemical medicine usually has many side effects, much worse than natural remedies, and exercise is an effort for me. I gladly held onto the pills until my mother, Sarah, returned once again from abroad.

A few days after Sarah arrived, I woke up one morning before church and found that my whole face, especially my jaw, was distorted and pulling up on one side. It looked exactly like a stroke victim's symptoms, and I fully believed that I had suffered something similar to a mild stroke! Following my mother's advice, I took it slow for a while and put my job search on hold. I tried the anti-depressants and soon realized this was not the way to go; I became so laid back and relaxed that we started calling it my "Zombie mode," where I had no responsibilities or obligations. I just sat in a chair all day, talking about the situation. Always searching for alternatives and better outcomes, we found a homeopathy practice near my area. They had a tunnel machine, which, at the time, was used for much more severe motor-neuron diseases. This machine actually worked wonders for my balance and coordination. They also supplied me with a stem-enhancement supplement, which I believed was a much-needed addition to my health regimen! I also started smoking again to stay as calm as possible. I rationalized this decision by noting that I suffered three setbacks during the six months I had quit smoking, and a bi-monthly relapse was unacceptable to me. So, I slowly started rebuilding my life, trying to feel as normal as possible, even though I was always aware of the unwelcome presence in my brain.

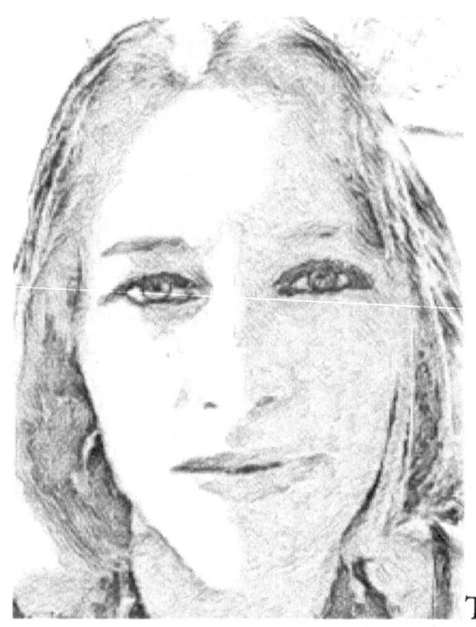

The thought that forever lurked in my mind was whether this condition called Multiple Sclerosis really existed. I often wondered quietly, but sometimes, I admitted these doubts aloud. I thought: Aren't these little things normal? Everyone sometimes loses their car keys, misses a step, gets lost on familiar roads, shivers when under pressure, or even gets those headaches where it feels like a clamp is squeezing their brain. Isn't this just me learning about the finer details of life?

The homeopath's tunnel machine was the same kind used on patients with much more aggressive, non-relapsing Multiple Sclerosis. It would start attacking your body and never stop, no matter what you did. So, I started using this machine, thinking that if Multiple Sclerosis really did exist, it would at least improve my condition. Together with the stem-enhancement therapy, my condition improved—I could now climb stairs without needing the railing for the first few steps, and I even managed some cartwheels on the grass with our children! I even convinced myself that the Multiple Sclerosis phenomenon might not really exist. I didn't know what a normal brain scan should look like, but I started thinking that the "milky way" we saw might just be the normal appearance of a skull for all I knew!

When it was time to say goodbye to Sarah again, I drove back to our flat with tears in my eyes but couldn't wait to return to our safe, quiet little nest. However, that same night, my peace was disrupted by the woman in the upstairs flat, who loved to walk around in high heels in the middle of the night. This was just the start of my dissatisfaction with our living quarters. Within a few days, things started to become really unpleasant. There were complaints about children playing outside their houses, and parents were instructed to keep their children inside. Was I supposed to raise my children in front of a TV screen? I was unhappy about this and felt the owners could invest in a play area for the children instead of parking spaces that were never used. My girls weren't the only children in the complex.

With the need to entertain and keep the girls indoors, the TV wasn't enough, so I bought an old-fashioned TV game console that Karin had pointed out to me. The girls and I had a lot of fun with it, but I still preferred them playing outside because that's what makes children truly happy and well-adjusted. With this in mind, I decided to get each of them a puppy. Now, we had three dogs, including my old lady, Pepper, who I'd had since just after high school. Soon after, I received a letter from the body corporate stating that the complex would now be a pet-free zone. No more pets allowed! There was no way I would abandon our pets, so I decided to give notice and move out of the place that had been our safe and quiet haven for years.

Thus began the search for a three-bedroom house with a big garden that was pet-friendly. It also needed to be safe, as I was a woman alone with two young girls, and it had to fit my budget. I firmly believed we would find the perfect place, and we did—a perfect three-bedroom house with a flat attached but with a separate entrance and small garden. An elderly couple lived there, and since our first meeting, they felt like family. Despite the house being on the corner of a busy intersection and having only a four-foot-high wall as a fence, my instincts told me this was it. I believed that locking up and protecting too much only made your property a bigger target for thieves. The busy traffic at the intersection would also deter criminals, as they would be noticed by motorists and passers-by. With Pearl's help, I started packing, and within a day of moving, everything was unpacked in our new home.

I hadn't been this happy or felt so secure, positive, and motivated in a long time. Everything fell into place one by one. I loved my neighbours; we never interfered in each other's lives, but we always had time for one another. My parents visited occasionally, and we all bonded like family.

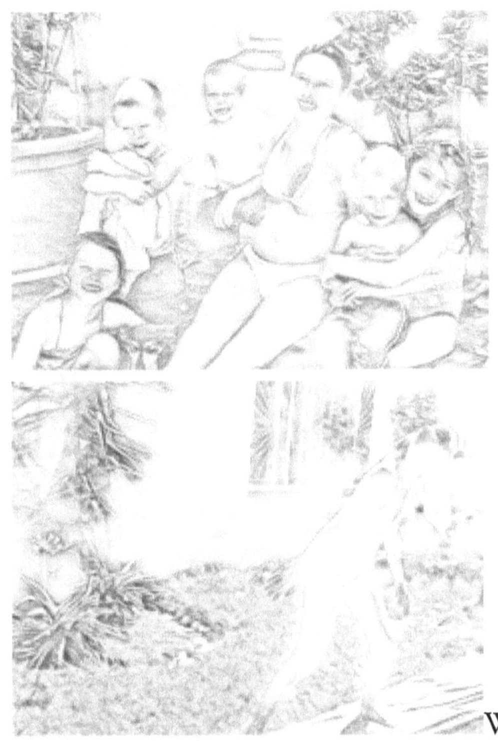

We had so much fun in that house. Even when Tjokkie, our youngest daughter's dog, would run away with one of our shoes or t-shirts, wagging his tail as if to say, "Catch me if you can!" These are the moments we still laugh about. There were sad times, too, like when Bella, our eldest daughter's dog, escaped the yard and ended up on the streets. We found her five days later, after searching and praying, at an SPCA we had already contacted. Despite Bella wearing a collar with my phone number on it, they had maintained she wasn't there! Thankfully, Karin's husband visited in person and found her. The joyful tears and emotions we experienced are unforgettable. This event made our house a place of joy, tears, and hard work. My father and I built a dog-proof addition to the fence to ensure none of the dogs would get out again.

After finishing a short course, I became a Payroll Certified Administrator (PCA). I felt I had proven to myself that I wasn't a "vegetable," even if only to myself. This qualification showed me I could still achieve my goals, drive in peak hour traffic, and overtake on a highway without problems. Yet, I still wasn't fully convinced and decided I needed more proof that I was still the same Marisa, unchanged by this unwelcome guest. I needed a bigger challenge, something I might have hesitated to do even before my diagnosis.

CHAPTER 3
COMBINING TALENTS

As I reflect on my various goals, I find it helpful to first identify them, assess which are realistic, and then determine how to turn the unrealistic ones into achievable objectives. While everyone's goals may differ, I believe we ultimately seek similar outcomes. My goals encompass: 1. Family life; 2. Financial success; 3. Soul calming; and 4. Health and wealth. Although health and wealth should ideally be prioritized, I feel that if I can stabilize the first three, the fourth will naturally follow.

I need to consider the resources available to me that can help achieve at least a 90% success rate in the first three areas. This seems to call for a strategic approach. Therefore, I will focus on the area where I perceive the least likelihood of reaching that success rate: financial success. Currently, my financial stability relies heavily on family support, giving me a 90% success rate. However, without this assistance, my self-sufficiency drops to about 20%. I anticipate that completing my degree will raise my self-sufficiency to 70%, and with dedication and hard work, I can eventually reach that 90% mark. But to do so, I must keep my "unwelcome guest" in check, as it poses challenges that could hinder my progress.

From an employer's perspective, the moment they learn about my medical condition, they may assume I'm desperate for work and might offer only a minimal salary, barely covering my transportation costs. I had to weigh whether it's worth it to disclose my condition on my resume. The positive aspects of my qualifications—such as education and references—often go unrecognized, despite proof that my condition is under control. My plan is to let my work speak for itself before introducing my unwelcome guest. There is always a risk of immediate dismissal for not disclosing a potentially impactful fact, so I must prepare for any outcome.

When it comes to family and friends, I feel confident that I'm already achieving close to a 90% success rate. By understanding their needs and being present for them, I foster an environment where they strive to understand me in return.

With one of my four goals already in the 90% range, I have strategies in place for the remaining two. For financial success, I just need to stay focused and committed. The third goal, soul calming, deserves more attention and dedication before I can see the benefits in health and wealth.

Interestingly, we discovered why our next-door neighbours feel like family. The uncle next door and my partner's father used to sing together in their youth, creating a connection that enhances our sense of

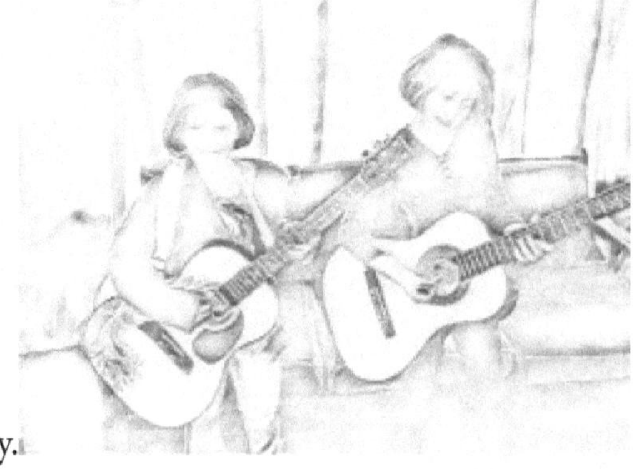

community.

We have a perfect patio for an arts and crafts studio, providing a quiet workspace away from the rush of daily life. This could serve as a fallback plan if my initial goal of returning to an office job doesn't work out.

I envision working on four clients' books while keeping an eye on my daughters as they complete their homework. With Pearl helping around the house, I no longer stress about keeping everything perfect. As I work on my art, the neighbour's uncle plays music from his studio, creating an inspiring atmosphere for creativity.

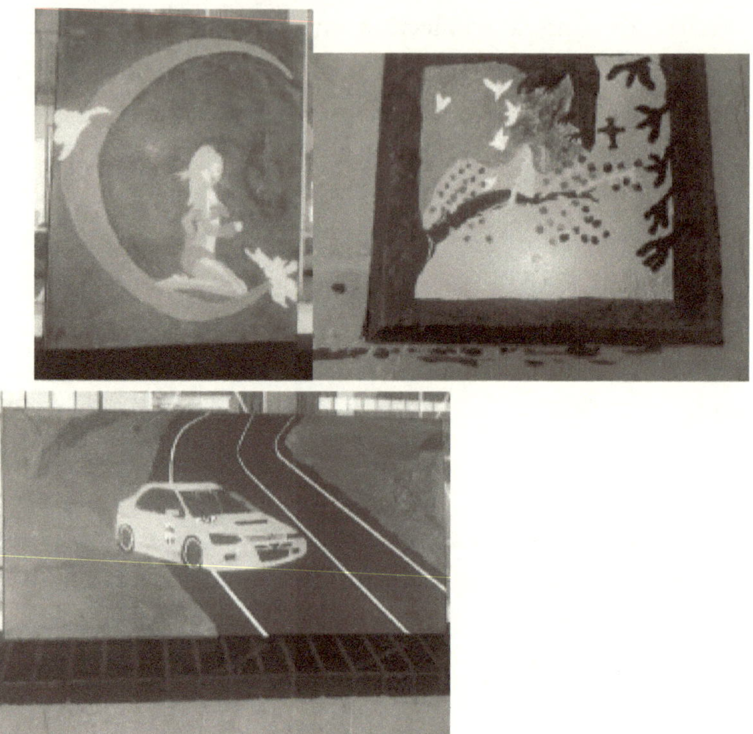

While I don't currently see my arts and crafts as marketable, I value them as a hobby and as gifts—nothing compares to a handmade present, which holds more meaning than a store-bought item.

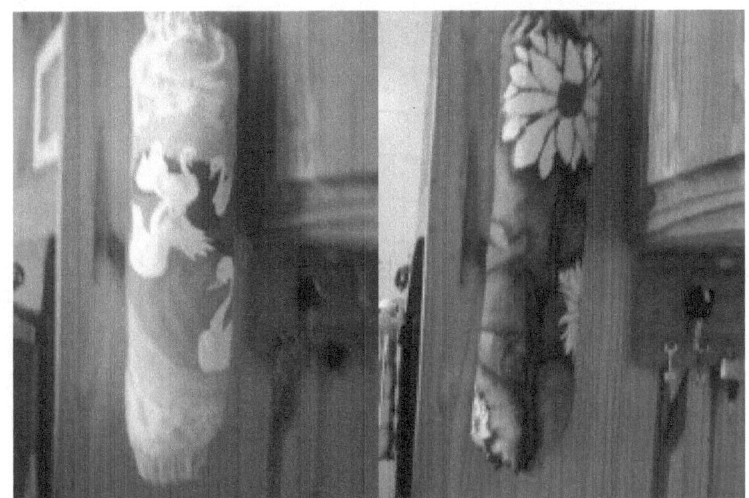

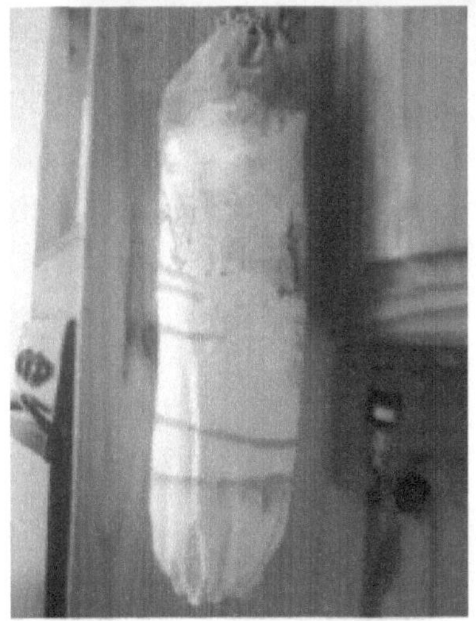

The girls enjoy crafting projects with me, and I cherish these moments. We display their artwork around our home, filling our space with warmth and love, even in the absence of their father.

I'm eagerly anticipating my parents' upcoming visit, counting down the days until we can share goodnight in person rather than through a screen. I also have an MRI scan scheduled during their stay for a routine check-up.

Fortunately, I've found a more compassionate neurologist who genuinely cares about her patients' well-being. Recent results showed no new relapses, only remnants of my first attack three years ago, motivating me to focus on my degree and kick-start my career.

However, despite everything falling into place, something feels missing. I've begun listening to my daughters about their emotional needs beyond physical support. They have what they need in terms of food, clothes, and medical care, but they long for more engagement with their father. Our youngest wishes for us to move to a place with horses, while the elder dreams of pursuing modelling and acting rather than just attending classes.

I won't make finding a permanent father figure a priority. My life is already full, and I can enjoy dinner dates now and then, which gives the girls a chance for restaurant meals. I am following my neurologist's prescription for Betaferon, which has stabilized my condition, although it comes with side effects.

The most challenging aspect for me has been dealing with injection marks on my body. For someone who didn't have stretch marks after two pregnancies, this is a significant adjustment. I've started wearing full-body swimsuits to cover the worst of the marks, but I'm gradually embracing my body, confident enough to wear a bikini during our next visit to the local pool. I plan to spend time in the cafeteria with friends while keeping an eye on my daughters as they play.

Despite concerns about potential cancer risks associated with Betaferon, our family history has been clear of such issues. To be safe, I eventually obtained a cancer policy.

The side effects of Betaferon also include increased appetite and a longing for physical touch. While these challenges are present, they don't overshadow my focus on more important aspects of life.

I find myself incorporating various strategies to keep the unwelcome guest at bay, whether it's through supplements, swimming, jogging, or yoga classes. I remain committed to all these activities as I work toward my ultimate goals of health and wealth.

As my final exams approach, I visited my GP for a cortisone prescription to help manage stress. I used to deny the stress associated with exams, but now I recognize its impact. Once my exam cycle ends, I won't seek another prescription, as cortisone has significant side effects, and I believe it should only be used cautiously.

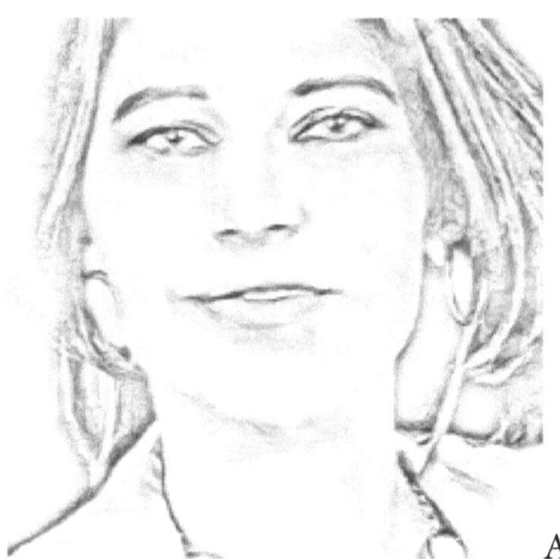

After completing my degree—a Bachelor of Business Administration in finance along with payroll certification—I wonder how my medical condition could still be a barrier, given my track record of stability. I plan to be honest about my condition on my resume, as employers cannot discriminate against employees with medical challenges.

I send out my resume daily, averaging two interviews a month. Given my circumstances, this isn't a bad rate. I have a letter from my neurologist confirming my ability to work full time in an office, despite some difficulties with stairs. After each interview, I leave filled with enthusiasm, yet I often hear nothing further. I continue serving my private clients after hours, even if I secure a permanent position.

I believe my time will come; I just need to be prepared and persistent. I hold onto the hope of finding an employer who sees my condition as just one aspect of who I am rather than my defining feature. I strive to achieve my dreams, viewing my medical condition merely as a temporary obstacle.

After months of searching, I found myself doubting whether an employer would truly understand and support my potential. I began to consider concealing my condition to let my abilities shine without the weight of my identity as a patient. This approach, while challenging, feels like the only way for my true potential to be recognized.

Whenever I sense sadness creeping in, I channel my energy into painting, playing with my daughters, or taking walks with our dogs. Despite the frustrations of job searching, I remind myself that the right opportunity will come along in due time. It may take longer than I hoped, but I'm committed to focusing on what I can control—my arts and crafts, my four accounting clients, and my search for employment. I even started putting out advertisements for new clients, but the response has mostly come from individuals seeking jobs with me.

Recognizing this, I've decided to stick with my current four clients. My resume is circulating on job sites, and I trust that potential employers will reach out. For now, I'm embracing the idea of letting opportunities come to me rather than actively searching. In the meantime, I'm exploring my creativity through making resin curtain binders and painted plastic bag holders. I believe there's always a way to continue moving forward on this journey.

CHAPTER 4
RENEW TALENTS

Our parents returned home, dragging their enormous suitcases that seemed to spell out 'warning: trouble ahead.' They informed us that their contracts abroad had not been renewed and that they were back for good this time—no more leaving. That first night, we didn't fully unpack or discuss our plans for what to do next. Instead, we chose to simply enjoy being together again.

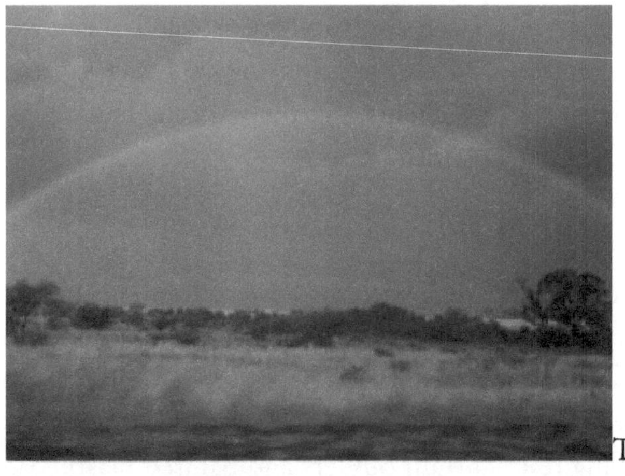

The next day, we finally faced the inevitable "what next" conversation, where everyone had their own opinions. I started by sharing my ideas and recommendations, knowing that my parents already had an idea of what I would suggest. They were well aware of my goals and limitations. I proposed that we focus on making art and craft products to sell, advertising them both online and at the yearly festival.

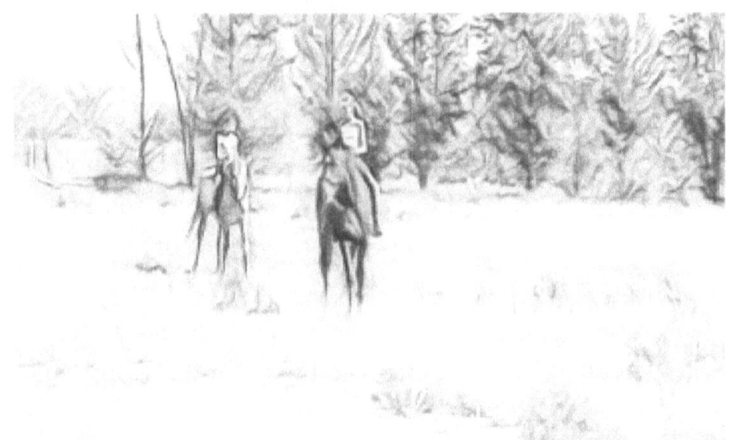

Meanwhile, the girls could enjoy some free horseback riding, which would create a peaceful, calming atmosphere.

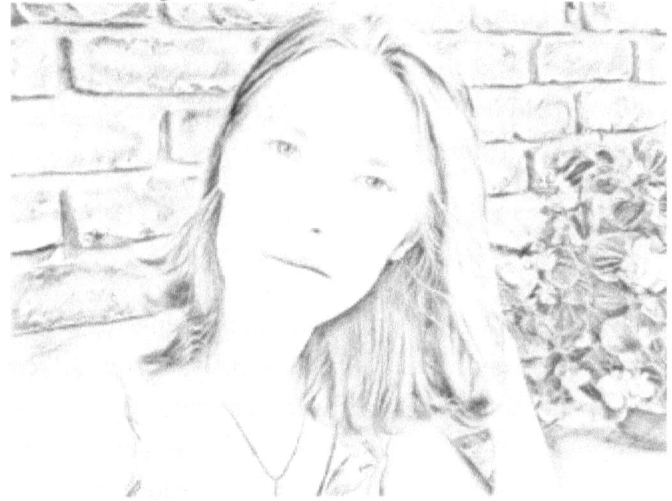

In that moment, I felt hopeful—genuinely hopeful. A rare clarity flooded my heart. The rainbow was more than just a beautiful scene; it was a symbol, a beacon of the life I wished to create for myself in this town, with its peacefulness and charm. I could almost feel my dream coming into focus.

But just as quickly, the warmth that filled my heart began to fade. The conversation in the car, once filled with excitement about Orania, shifted back to reality—Burgersfort. It felt like my hope, so tangible just moments before, was being quietly taken away. As my parents spoke of practicalities, Burgersfort became the topic that dominated, and I could feel my confidence draining. The rainbow, the clarity, the dreams—it all slipped away. What had felt like a promise now seemed like a distant, unattainable fantasy, and the weight of it settled over me like a shadow. The unwelcome guest crept in again, silently tallying another point on its scoreboard.

Final outcomes were usually discouraging. I felt like I was hitting a wall, and the hope that started to grow was slowly being chipped away with each rejection. I understood that people judged my abilities based on what they could see physically—without knowing the fire that still burned inside me to contribute, to work, and to prove that my illness didn't define me.

But through this challenging period, I kept reminding myself of the bigger picture. I had to stay focused on what truly mattered: keeping my family together, adapting to new surroundings, and maintaining my health and mental well-being, no matter what professional setbacks I faced. The warmth of my family and the sense of purpose they gave me were far more valuable than any fleeting success I might achieve in a career.

The transition to Burgersfort became a turning point for me. It forced me to reconcile my ambitions with the reality of living with a chronic illness. I couldn't continue to pretend I was just like everyone else. I had to embrace my limitations as part of my identity, not as something to be ashamed of, but as something that shaped me into the person I had become.

Despite the frustrations, I knew that this was just another chapter in the journey I had been on since the unwelcome guest entered my life. Every change, every loss, and every moment of joy or sadness had helped me become stronger. And no matter what, I would keep going—finding new ways to renew my talents and passions, adjusting to whatever came next.

Ultimately, my journey isn't just about surviving, but thriving, even when the odds seem stacked against me. And that's a lesson worth living for.

CHAPTER 5
LESS DEPRESSION

As we already know, work can multiply life's stress levels, but depression is especially dangerous. Being unemployed with no income makes depression bolder, giving the unwelcome guest a huge, undeserved advantage.

When we arrived at our three-bedroom house late that night, we were greeted by the warm glow of lights from the bedroom window. Despite the late hour, we were full of energy, eager to unpack and settle in. The next morning, with the sun streaming in, we were thrilled to discover just how lovely the house was—a cozy, comfortable three-bedroom home with everything we needed. And as a delightful bonus, there were twelve magnificent horses! It felt like we had found a hidden treasure, and we were determined to make the best of our new beginning. My parents and I were perfectly content, though the girls were a bit less excited. They had hoped for something as polished and glamorous as their friends' homes.

Our girls soon found joy in helping with the horses. Zans, our youngest, would be up at the crack of dawn, eager to help with the morning feedings. It was clear that she had found her calling—she was captivated by the world of horses. What began as a dream of becoming a show jumper soon evolved into a fascination with horse philosophy, breeding, and health. Meanwhile, our eldest, Tina, continued to pursue her dreams of modelling and acting. Both girls were chasing their passions, and while wealthier parents might have smoothed their path, we knew that love, family, and support were even more valuable. We wanted to inspire them to carve out their own futures, filled with the joy of pursuing their dreams.

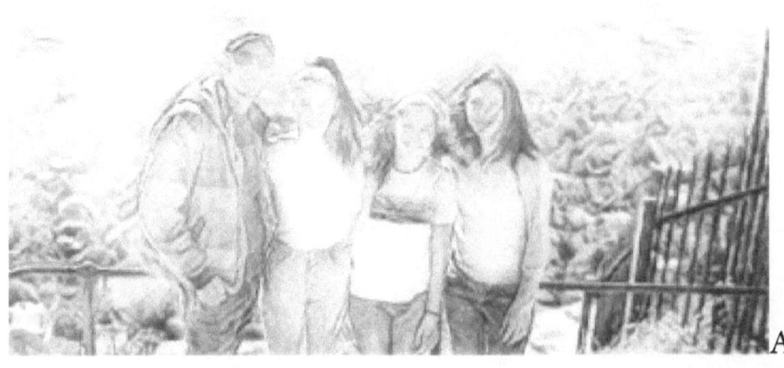

As for me, I was excited to rebuild my career, and Jaco was ready to shift his focus from the Vaal Triangle to the East Rand. I've come to realize that life often happens while you're making plans, but I was confident that everything would work out in the end.

Within just three months, we had moved from Burgersfort back to Benoni, where everything was ready for us—our home, schooling for the girls, and even our transport was all arranged. Through hard work, grace, and a bit of luck, everything had fallen into place. I felt optimistic about our future. Benoni offered even more opportunities, and I knew I could expand my client base and reconnect with old ones more easily.

In the meantime, my father and I took on jobs at a local real estate agency, thanks to the support from our church's care group. The girls quickly settled back into their old school, and their primary school welcomed them with open arms—no complications, just a smooth transition. It felt like everything was falling into place.

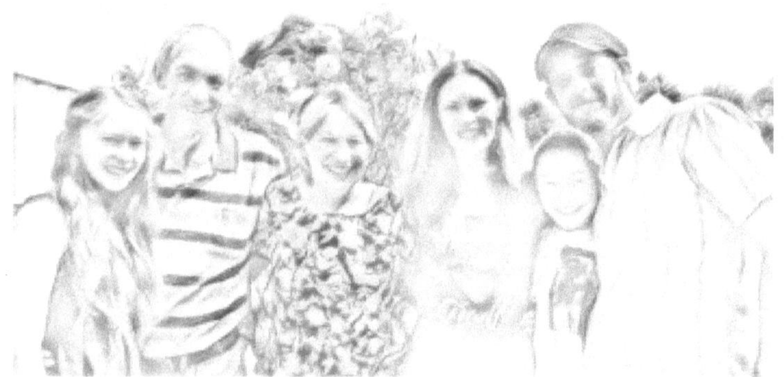

Over the festive season, Jaco came to stay with us. He was there to help with the girls, but his presence brought so much more—laughter, joy, and love filled the house from morning till night. I hadn't realized just how much I missed him until then. His warmth and humour were a constant source of happiness. I knew that as long as we stayed together, we could handle anything.

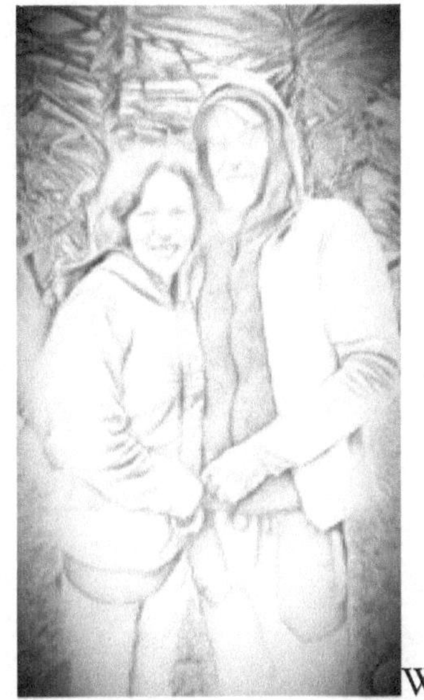

When the opportunity came to move back to Jaco in our hometown, I made the choice to stay and keep building what we had started in the East Rand. At the time, it felt like the right decision, though we would later see it differently. But for now, I was focused on gaining more experience and building myself up. My job had been good to us, and both my parents and Jaco were employed with the same company. Things seemed to be going well—until the day the company announced it was shutting down. No more secure income or "pizza Fridays." We found ourselves back at square one, searching for new opportunities.

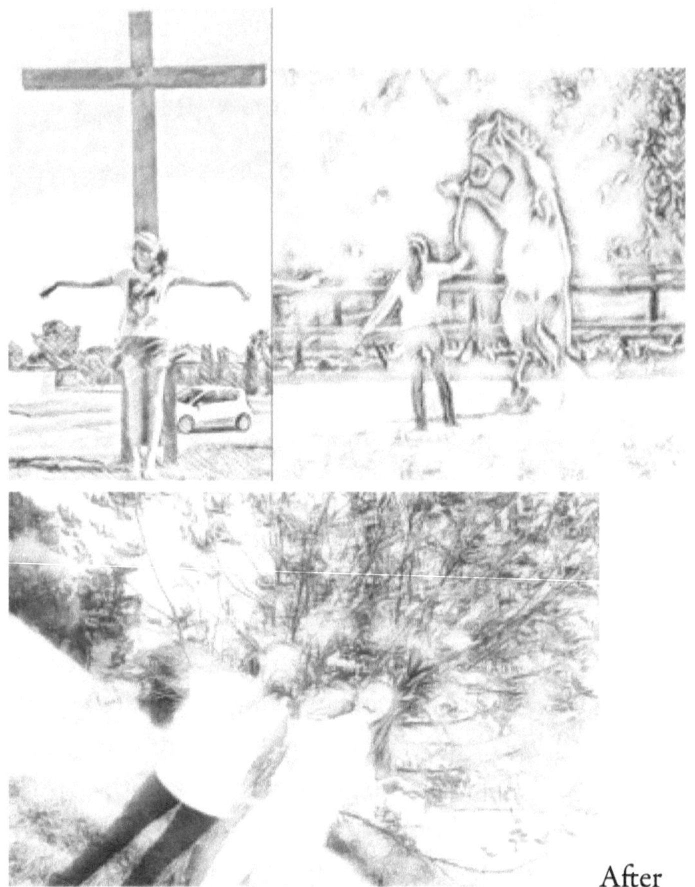

After I finally moved through the heaviest period of mourning, Jaco picked me up, and together, we decided to repair the beautiful marriage that I had once, in a moment of heartache, let slip away. Now, with my heart aching to regain everything I lost, we began planning our second wedding—this time, an intimate celebration with only our closest family.

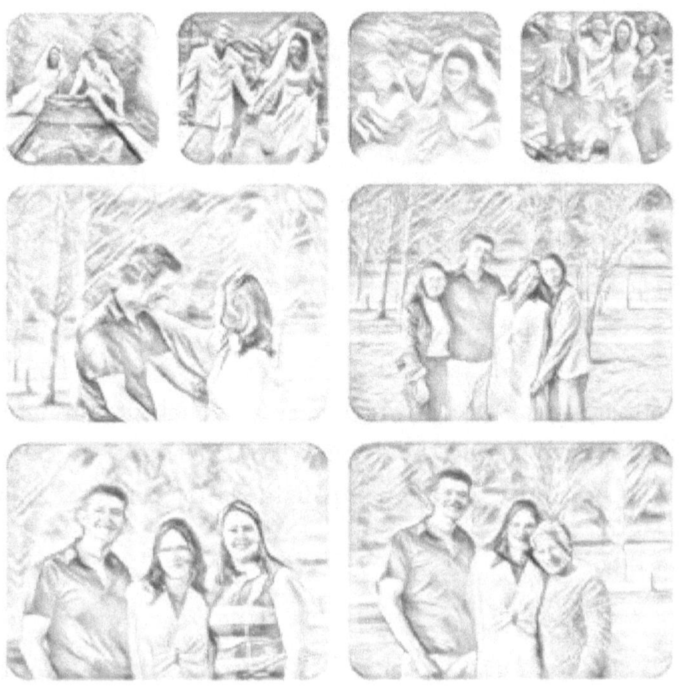

CHAPTER 6
SOLO

This is how it felt being without my husband by my side. I'm surrounded by love and people who care, but nothing fills the space of the fulfilment we share when Jaco and I face life together. Though there's no actual war, it feels like an internal battle—a war of words within me, a clash between cells. Jaco dreams of working abroad to provide fully for our family. I support him in making this dream a reality, even though the thought of him leaving fills me with fear. He helps me walk, keeps me on track with my exercises, and holds me steady in this fight against my unwelcome guest.

We quickly devised a plan and a budget to make this dream possible, which included selling my car—no longer an option for me to drive medically. Half of my retrenchment package, along with support from Jaco's sister, Ogies, helped set the foundation. Every day spent planning and packing his bags just felt wrong, but I knew I had to be strong, to support my husband in the way he's always supported me, no matter the tears or the aching absence I would feel.

I've battled this illness before and managed to work through it, but now, without medical aid, I have to keep a stable, stress-free environment while Jaco arranges for me to eventually join him abroad. Together, we strategized that this path might offer better opportunities for us, given how elusive decent employment in South Africa has been. Every interview felt like it was "the one," only to end in disappointment and silence. It's disheartening.

The house, full of people, always felt empty without my partner there. Jaco not only helps me with the day-to-day routines but also keeps me calm, helping to minimize the stress and depression that often follow. I've had to learn to

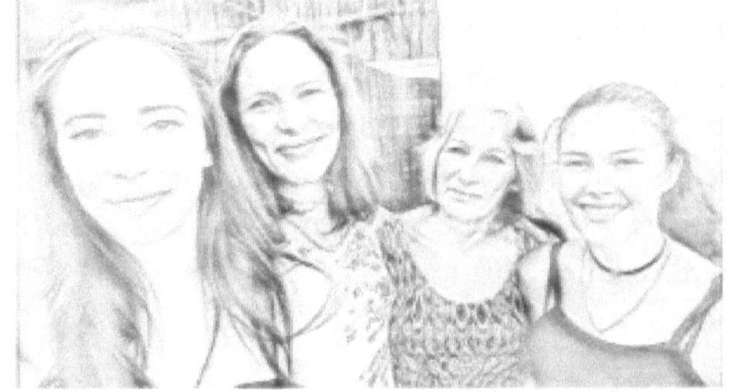

tackle chores again as the "old Marisa" once did, but each time I stumbled, it only made the tasks harder to complete. Our household was filled with female energy—my mother, our two daughters, and me. We divided the chores according to everyone's schedule; I took charge of the laundry since I could start early and finish later in the day. On laundry-free days, I'd do a quick exercise routine, dress up completely, makeup and all, just to tend the garden, plant seeds, or pull weeds.

One day, I managed the laundry without any trouble, but as I took the clothes off the line, my left knee suddenly froze. My leg wouldn't move forward at all. I called out to my mother, but she was absorbed in her reading and didn't hear me. The girls were at work, and it was just me and our four dogs in the yard. I instructed my little Yorkshire terrier, Rocky, to get my mother's attention, and bless him, he was quick to alert her. Without Rocky, I might have had to yell loud enough for the entire neighbourhood or resort to crawling back to the house.

Independence was a core value for me from a young age, but life has now reshaped that identity, urging me to accept reliance as part of my journey. This is the hand I've been dealt, perhaps one of life's lessons before I can fulfil my dreams. I maintain a semblance of independence—I am, after all, the lessee of our rented home—even if it's limited to washing dishes or waiting in the car while others shop for us. I pace my errands early in the day, before the heat drains me, to conserve energy and manage spending. With discipline in our finances, I could join Jaco in Scotland and perhaps find better treatment options. I might even work again, like many couples do there, building a life together.

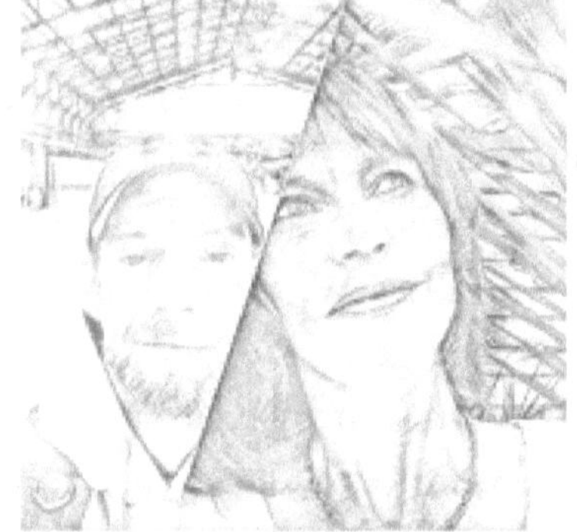

But reality shifted again when we received shocking news: I might not be granted entry into the UK. Then came the tragic news of Jaco's sister's passing, bringing him home for the funeral—a heartbreaking return. Her passing gave us pause, a time to reassess our plans. I trust that God's plans are far better than anything I could imagine, guiding us through these challenges with purpose.

With the girls now living independently, we're simplifying life, applying for jobs again in hopes of rebuilding our lives here. I try to keep faith through every interview, but the constant lack of responses chips away at my confidence. I've always been qualified, experienced, and driven, and Jaco has the determination of ten people. Yet, the struggles mount.

We made the tough decision to sell our only car, as its repair costs outweighed its usefulness. Our belongings, too, were pared down to the essentials—a bed, a stove—as we prepared for a more modest lifestyle. Our landlord offered us a smaller unit, but it came with one condition: no pets. Our three dogs had been like family, each with a piece of our hearts. Thankfully, a friend across the road offered to care for them, but it broke our hearts to hear their cries every time we visited.

Our one-bedroom unit felt stifling, boxed in by the complex's dumpsters, with walls that absorbed every ounce of heat. Though Jaco assisted the landlords with maintenance in lieu of rent, the setup was far from ideal. It was unbearably hot and cramped, with our belongings stacked to the ceiling. I often thought of how I'd love just one more lap around an ice rink, a reminder of life's cycles. Each loop, like life's hardships, is softened by knowing that the end of one journey is merely the beginning of another.

The cycles of joy, sadness, love, and frustration mirror our relationships. Sometimes love feels easy; other times, it's a constant effort. I've learned to give myself the silent treatment when frustration bubbles up, holding back words that might sting, knowing they'd leave a mark. This unwelcome guest in my life may be relentless, but it will never have the last word. I have days when running away seems tempting, but I know the guest would follow. In every family portrait, we look so happy, yet inside, I feel fractured. Why can't I just be myself again? Why can't this "parasite" find someone else to haunt?

Even in my darkest moments, I know I'll keep pushing forward. Life may challenge me, but it doesn't get to define me. This story isn't over; I refuse to let this condition be the closing chapter. On my hardest days, I hold onto those glimmers of the real me, the part that shines even when hidden. Every step forward is a victory, a reminder of the strength I have to reclaim my life.

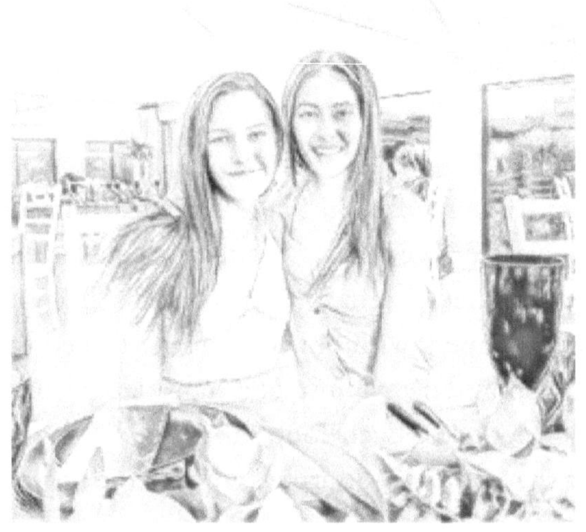

One evening, Jaco and I discussed what might help ease the strain: a simpler, slower pace. We decided to return to our hometown, a place where stress wouldn't hinder my focus on recovery. I know I have the strength within me, and maybe, just maybe, life isn't done showing me what I'm capable of.

The next morning, an unexpected call came. A company wanted Jaco to join their team, with enough support to secure us a pet-friendly apartment in the Vaal Triangle. It felt as though a door had finally opened. Moving back to our roots, where I could access chronic medication and regain stability, became our next step. Our friend who had kept our dogs agreed to help transport us back, along with our belongings and our beloved pets. And though we arrived a week past Jaco's intended start date, the day felt perfect. Our dogs, reunited with us, seemed as relieved and happy as we were.

CHAPTER 7
CONCLUSION

Is this the new Marisa, back in the old town where everything inside me began to evolve? Had I stayed here, perhaps I would have found this sense of peace, health, and clarity years ago. But I fought against it, refusing to let go of the Marisa I had always known. Now, I am Marisa with my unwelcome guest. I realize now that MS does not define me; it is simply a part of my life that I've come to understand and accept. "Aim for the moon; if you miss, you'll be among the stars." I truly understand this now. Find your stars—both the positive and the negative—and work until even the negative aligns with your inner light.

On days I cleaned the house, I often fell, and one day, the neighbour rushed in to help me up. She encouraged me with kind words, reminding me of my strength and positivity, and said I was an inspiration to her. It blessed me deeply to know that my struggles could inspire others. At home, Jaco and I spend time keeping our apartment tidy, planning time with friends, and savouring each moment. But just before New Year's, I found myself in the hospital with an unexpected complication. My skin had turned yellow, and the doctor advised an emergency trip to the hospital if it didn't clear up. Even though yellow is my favourite colour, I didn't want my skin to match it.

One evening, Jaco returned home and saw that I could barely stand. He quickly called the ambulance, and our neighbours gathered with encouragement and prayers as I was taken to Sebokeng Hospital. The paramedics were kind, assuring me they'd take me somewhere I could get help. I arrived to see a crowded waiting room and felt fortunate to be admitted so quickly. Seeing everyone waiting, I felt a mix of compassion and hope that I might finally get the referral needed for chronic MS care. We opened Christmas gifts on my hospital bed, grateful for each other's presence. Two days later, I was discharged with a treatment plan and instructions to follow up at a neurology centre.

We celebrated New Year's with friends as planned, surrounded by people who understood my challenges and helped me move freely. I shared my hopes and worries about the upcoming hospital visit, nervous but hopeful. A few days later, Jaco accompanied me to the appointment at Baragwanath Hospital. After waiting through long queues, I finally met with a neurologist. She reviewed my MRI scans and explained where the MS scars appeared, adding me to the waiting list for chronic medication.

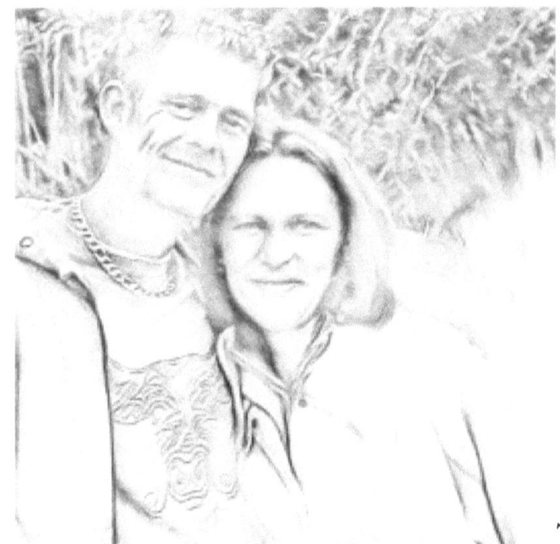

The waiting felt endless, but friends like Peter and Jené supported me. Peter offered to help publish this book, and Jené recommended natural remedies to strengthen my veins and ease my MS symptoms. Coconut oil, B vitamins, magnesium, and other supplements could help—but I could only wait, hoping that soon I'd get access to the resources I needed.

Some nights I lay awake, memories of my first MS attack flashing through my mind. Back then, it was easier to find medical care and employment, with a car and city conveniences nearby. Now, my path felt different but no less meaningful. As I wait for the call that could open new doors, I dream of rejoining the workforce, contributing, and balancing my time between work, family, and friends.

After all, finding the real Marisa took a long journey through pain, depression, and resilience. I fought hard to hold onto my identity, refusing to let go of everything "Marisa" meant to me. But now, I am not just Marisa. I am Marisa who lives with her unwelcome guest—not as my identity but as a testament to my journey and strength.

"Aim for the moon, and if you miss, you'll be among the stars." Find your, stars, know their light and shadows, and embrace the good. The words our girls were raised.

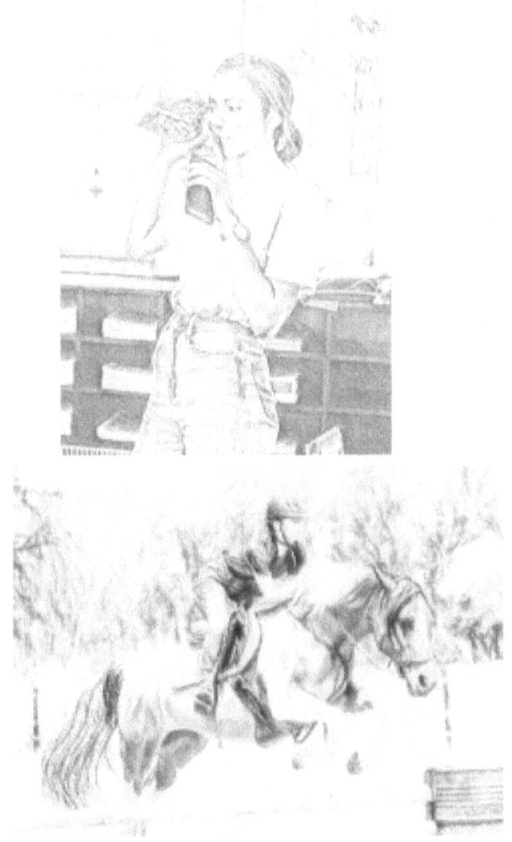

Work patiently with the darker moments until they, too, align with positivity. I'm grateful to everyone who believed in me and gave me a chance. Now, beyond the walls of my apartment, I look forward to new dreams, awaiting my call and the freedom to explore life once again.

In the heart of the bustling city, where skyscrapers kissed the sky, I was once a driven, professional woman climbing the corporate ladder. Now, confined by illness, I found myself redefining purpose beyond ambition. Though job interviews once felt like a way back to my old life, my worth now lies beyond titles or capabilities. With creativity, writing, and connection, I found purpose anew.

Though my journey diverged from what I once envisioned, I know it's far from over. Beyond the walls that once felt like a prison, endless possibilities await.

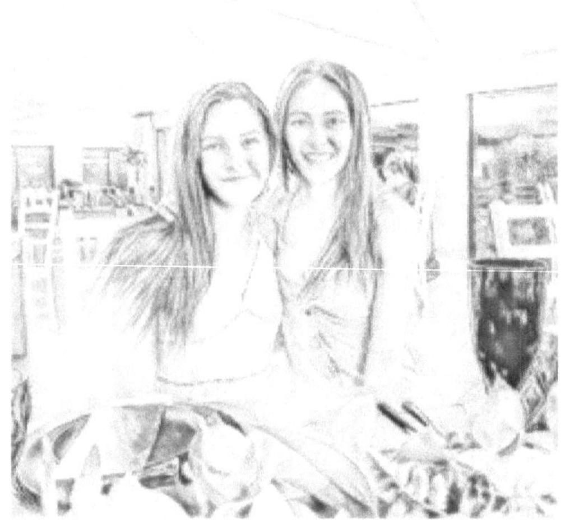

Through this whole ordeal, I learned that true strength reveals itself when there is no choice but to be strong. Support from family and friends has been invaluable, and, above all, I've learned that with God's hand, so much can be accomplished. Writing my story has given me an unexpected sense of inner peace, a healing that words—or even painting—could express.

Now, feeling ready to pursue a new chapter in a remote lifestyle while letting hobbies remain as hobbies, no 8-5 responsibilities, leaving me with time to make the 8-5 responsibilities taking care of the one thing that matters most for every instance, HEALTH. Concentrating on new 8-5 responsibilities including: Exercises, Meditation (which normally ends in prayer), Healthy food, Natural remedy use for fixing body from inside;

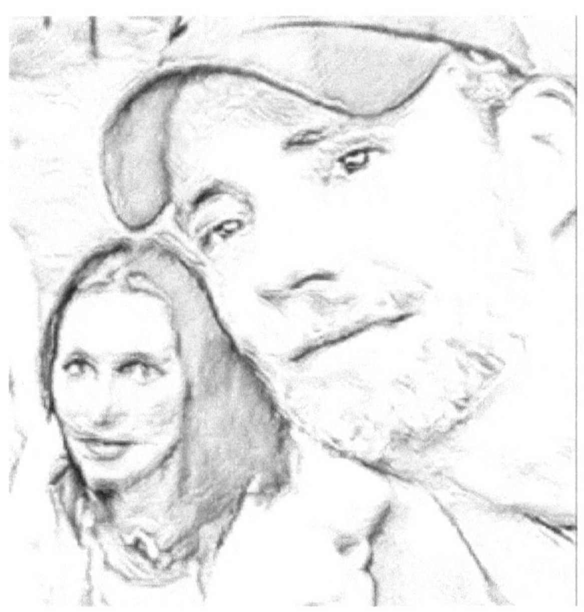

I want to extend my heartfelt thanks to ChatGPT and Varius Publishing. Your guidance in bringing this book to life is deeply appreciated, and it's my hope that these pages bring comfort, insight, and encouragement to every reader.

INDEX

Chapter	Name	Page
1	MEETING THE UNWELCOMED GUEST	1
2	CALM WATERS	46
3	COMBINING TALENTS	63
4	RENEW TALENTS	76
5	LESS DEPRESSION	82
6	SOLO	90
7	CONCLUSION	99

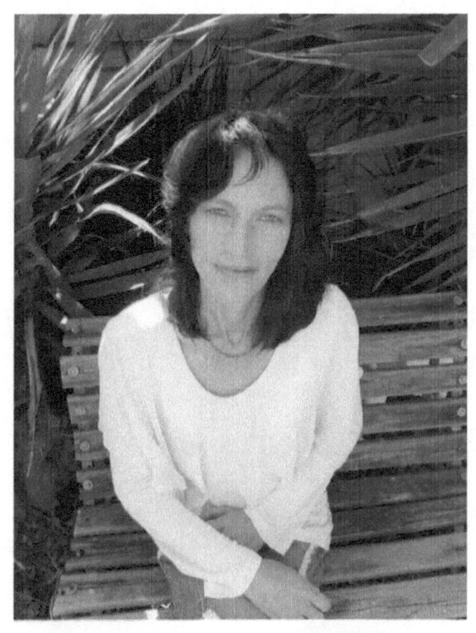

About the Author

The author is an ambitious and creative individual, driven by a strong sense of family orientation. Known for their polite and friendly demeanour, they approach life with a positive outlook and a genuine desire to connect with others.

Read more at https://www.facebook.com/ MATIZACREATIONS.